The Calm Mind Diet

How to Eat Your Way to Less Stress and More Happiness

By

Dwight W. Gagne

DISCLAIMER

Table Contents

Introduction

How Food Affects Your Mood

Have you ever reached for a bag of chips, a pint of ice cream, or a bottle of wine as a coping mechanism when you were feeling pressured, anxious, or depressed? Have you ever wondered how your eating habits impact your well-being, mental health, and mood? Then you are not by yourself. Emotional eating, mood swings, and mental health problems are common problems that many people face due to their dietary and lifestyle choices.

This book will teach you how eating can help you de-stress and how it influences your mood. You will learn the physiological underpinnings of stress and anxiety, as well as how they affect your hormones, gut, and brain. You will discover how probiotics can help balance your mood and enhance your mental health, as well as the link between the gut and the brain. Additionally, you will discover how an anti-inflammatory diet can strengthen your immune system, lower inflammation, and prevent brain deterioration.

Additionally, you will learn which foods to eat more of for a happy mind and which to avoid or restrict for a calmer mind. You will discover the benefits of herbs and spices, including how they can improve your mood and help you unwind. You will also learn about the significance of hydration and how to drink more water to stay healthy and hydrated. Additionally, you will discover how to reduce or completely cut out sugar, alcohol, and caffeine from your diet, as well as how they affect your mood.

You will also learn how to prepare and cook nutritious meals and snacks, as well as how to eat with awareness and enjoyment. Along with learning how to create a welcoming and encouraging eating environment, you will also learn how to manage cravings and emotional eating. Lastly, you will discover how to make a mental health eating action plan, monitor your development, and recognize your accomplishments.

You will know more about how food impacts your mood at the end of this book, and you will also know how to use food as a tool to enhance your mental and physical health. Along with enjoying the mental health advantages of eating, you will also know how to make mindful and healthy food choices. You'll experience an increase in self-assurance, vigor, and happiness in your life.

Are you prepared to go on your path to mental clarity and happiness? Now let's get started!

Chapter 1

The Science of Stress and Anxiety

Anxiety and stress are common emotions that have an impact on people's physical and mental well-being. Anxiety is a state of fear, worry, or nervousness, whereas stress is a reaction to a perceived threat or challenge. Numerous physiological and psychological changes, including elevated heart rate, blood pressure, tense muscles, perspiration, trouble breathing, and negative emotions, can be brought on by stress and anxiety. But not all anxiety and tension are bad. People can be inspired to perform better, handle difficulties, and conquer barriers by a certain amount of stress and anxiety. It's important to learn appropriate coping mechanisms for stress and anxiety to keep them from getting worse or overwhelming you.

Understanding how the body and brain respond to stressful and anxiety-inducing circumstances, as well as how these responses impact health and well-being, is central to the science of stress and anxiety. The hypothalamic-pituitary-adrenal (HPA) axis, which controls the release of stress hormones including cortisol and adrenaline, is one of the primary systems implicated in stress and anxiety. These hormones set up the body for the fight-or-flight reaction, a survival strategy that allows people to respond swiftly to potentially fatal circumstances. However, excessive or prolonged activation of the HPA axis can harm several organs and systems, including the neurological, immunological, digestive, and cardiovascular systems. The amygdala, a brain region involved in emotional processing and fear conditioning, and the hippocampus, a brain region involved in memory and learning, can both be negatively impacted by long-term stress and anxiety.

Cognitive and emotional issues like poor memory, focus, decision-making, mood regulation, and resilience may result from this.

Thankfully, there are lots of strategies to improve health and well-being while lowering stress and anxiety. The best tactics include progressive muscular relaxation, breathing exercises, yoga, meditation, and biofeedback, among other relaxation methods. These methods can help calm the nervous system, reduce stress hormone levels, and promote mindfulness and relaxation. Additional tactics include cognitive-behavioral therapy (CBT), a type of psychotherapy that teaches patients how to recognize and confront the unfavorable ideas and attitudes that fuel stress and anxiety, as well as how to swap them out for more practical and uplifting ones. Additionally,

CBT can assist individuals in acquiring coping mechanisms like assertiveness, problem-solving, and exposure to stressful situations. Lifestyle choices like consistent exercise, a balanced diet, enough sleep, social support, and engaging in hobbies can also help avoid and manage anxiety and stress by enhancing mental and physical health, elevating mood and self-esteem, and giving life meaning and purpose.

1. The Gut-Brain Connection and the Role of Probiotics

The network of communication between your gut and brain is known as the "gut-brain connection." There are numerous physiological and pharmacological connections between these two organs. Live microorganisms known as probiotics can positively impact the diversity and balance of your gut microbiota, thereby improving your gut health. Through their production of neurotransmitters, immune system modulation, and vagus nerve interaction, they may also have an impact on the health of your brain.

Probiotics may aid in enhancing mental health, mood, and cognitive performance, according to certain research. They might also change the gut-brain axis, which would lessen stress, anxiety, and depression.

To fully comprehend the mechanics and impacts of probiotics on the gut-brain axis, as well as the best probiotic kinds and dosages for various circumstances, more research is necessary.

Here's a little poem I wrote about probiotics and the gut-brain connection:

The brain and the stomach communicate constantly.

They affect each other's health and function by exchanging signals, chemicals, and information.

They create a dynamic and intricate intersection.

Probiotics are beneficial bacteria that reside in the stomach and can support the immune system and gut flora.

They may also have a variety of effects on the brain.

They can control stress and release neurotransmitters.

The gut-brain axis may benefit from probiotic use.

They might enhance mental health, mood, and cognitive function, but further studies are required to fully validate these benefits.
and to determine whether probiotics are ideal in various situations.

2.The Anti-Inflammatory Diet and Its Benefits for Mental Health

The goal of the anti-inflammatory diet is to lessen inflammation in the body, which has been connected to several chronic illnesses and mental health issues. This is a succinct explanation of the anti-inflammatory diet and its potential advantages for improving mental health:
The anti-inflammatory diet is a broad guideline that emphasizes eating more fruits, vegetables, whole grains, healthy fats, herbs, and spices; it is not a strict or

rigid plan. Instead, it limits or avoids foods that may cause inflammation, such as processed foods, refined sugars, red meat, alcohol, and other foods.

The immune system uses inflammation as a normal and healthy defense mechanism against allergies, wounds, and infections. On the other hand, persistent or severe inflammation can harm healthy cells and tissues and be a contributing factor in several health concerns, including cancer, diabetes, Alzheimer's disease, and cardiovascular disease.

Because chronic inflammation can disrupt the synthesis and operation of neurotransmitters, which are chemical messengers that control emotions, thoughts, and behavior, it can also have an impact on mood and the brain. The stress response system, which can result in anxiety, sadness, and other mental health problems, can also be triggered by inflammation.

By offering essential nutrients, antioxidants, and phytochemicals that can shield the brain from oxidative stress and inflammation and promote the production and function of neurotransmitters, an anti-inflammatory diet may help enhance mental health. These nutrients include, but are not limited to, polyphenols, magnesium, zinc, folate, vitamin B12, and omega-3 fatty acids.

A healthy gut microbiome, or the assemblage of bacteria and other microorganisms that reside in the digestive tract, may be supported by an anti-inflammatory diet. Through the gut-brain axis, a bidirectional communication network that links the immunological, endocrine, and neurological systems, the gut microbiota can affect mood and mental health. Beneficial compounds that help regulate inflammation and mood, such as serotonin and short-chain fatty acids, are produced by a diverse and well-balanced gut microbiota.

The DASH diet and the Mediterranean diet, two well-known eating regimens that have been demonstrated to improve both physical and mental health, are comparable to the anti-inflammatory diet. The anti-inflammatory diet is a supportive and preventive approach that can improve general health and quality of life, rather than a treatment for any illness or condition.

3.Foods to Avoid or Limit for a Calmer Mind

Stress is a prevalent issue in the demanding and fast-paced world of today. It may impact our performance, well-being, and attitude. While there are numerous strategies to manage stress, including physical activity, mindfulness, and relaxation methods, our food is frequently disregarded. Stress levels and mental health can be significantly impacted by the foods we eat. While certain foods might help us feel less stressed and anxious, others can make them worse. For a peaceful mind, limit or stay away from these meals.

- Red meats. Saturated fat, cholesterol, and salt levels are elevated in red meats, particularly those that are processed. These may raise blood pressure, oxidative stress, and inflammation in the body, which may cause the stress hormone cortisol to be released. Cortisol can affect mood, memory, and cognitive abilities. Additionally, red foods are heavy in iron, which can build up in the brain and harm neurons through oxidative stress. High red meat consumption has been associated with a higher incidence of anxiety and depression. You should only consume red meat three times a week, and if you do, go for lean or grass-fed cuts.

- Margarine sticks and butter. Saturated fats, including butter and stick margarine, can increase inflammation and cholesterol. Additionally, they include trans fats, which are synthetic lipids that can raise bad cholesterol (LDL) and decrease good cholesterol (HDL). Additionally, trans fats may hinder the synthesis of serotonin, a neurotransmitter that controls appetite, mood, and sleep. Anxiety, irritation, and depression can result from low serotonin levels. When possible, steer clear of butter and stick to margarine in favor of healthy substitutes like nut butter, avocados, and olive oil.

- cheeses. Cheeses taste great, but they can also cause mental tension. Tyramine, an amino acid found in high concentrations in cheeses, can release norepinephrine, another stress hormone. Blood pressure, heart rate, and alertness can all rise when norepinephrine is released, which can exacerbate anxiety and restlessness. Additionally, casein, a protein found in cheese, can bind to the brain and create opiates, which can lead to addiction and withdrawal symptoms. Cheeses may also contain significant levels of sodium, which can cause fluid retention and blood pressure to rise. Eat no more than one ounce of cheese each day, and choose aged or low-fat types as they contain less casein and tyramine.

- sweets and pastries. Sweets and pastries are delicious, but they may also be bad for your brain. Refined sugar, which is abundant in pastries and sweets, can cause blood glucose levels to rise and fall. This may have an impact on how well the brain uses glucose as fuel, which may have negative effects on mood, memory, and cognitive performance. Additionally, sugar can cause the production of insulin, which in turn can reduce dopamine and serotonin levels—two neurotransmitters that are linked to motivation and happiness. In addition to causing oxidative stress

and inflammation, sugar can also
damage brain tissue and raise the
risk of neurodegenerative illnesses.
Try to limit your intake of pastries
and sweets; instead, indulge in
fruits, dark chocolate, or honey to
satisfy your sweet craving.

- Fast food or fried food. Fast food
  and fried foods may be handy, but
  they may also be bad for the brain.
  Fast food and fried foods are heavy
  in calories, fat, salt, and additives,
  which can raise blood pressure,
  cholesterol, and inflammation.
  Additionally, they may lessen
  blood flow to the brain, which may
  compromise oxygen delivery and
  function. The bacteria that inhabit
  the digestive tract, known as the
  gut microbiome, can be impacted
  by fried or fast food. The
  neurological, endocrine, and
  immunological systems are linked

via the gut-brain axis, a communication network that allows the gut microbiota to affect brain function and behavior. Beneficial compounds that can enhance mood and brain function include vitamins, neurotransmitters, and short-chain fatty acids, which can be produced by a healthy gut microbiota. Upset gut flora can produce hazardous compounds, including lipopolysaccharides, ammonia, and toxins, that can pass across the blood-brain barrier and induce oxidative stress and inflammation in the brain. To support the health of your gut microbiome, limit your intake of fried and fast food and increase your intake of probiotic and prebiotic foods, including yogurt, kefir, sauerkraut, bananas, oats, and garlic.

In summary, our stress levels and mental health can be greatly impacted by the foods we eat. While certain foods might help us feel less stressed and anxious, others can make them worse. We can achieve a calmer mind and a healthier body by avoiding or limiting foods that can harm the brain, like red meats, butter and stick margarine, cheeses, pastries and sweets, and fried or fast food, and by eating more foods that can benefit the brain, like whole grains, green leafy vegetables, berries, nuts, beans, fish, poultry, olive oil, and wine.

Chapter 2

Foods to Eat More of for a Happier Mind

In addition to being a mental state, happiness is also influenced by our diet. There are several ways in which our food might affect our mental, emotional, and cognitive health. Certain meals can give us vital nutrients, antioxidants, and phytochemicals that improve the health and function of our brains. To have a happier mind, increase your intake of these meals.

fatty seafood: Omega-3 fatty acids, which are essential for maintaining brain function, are abundant in fatty fish, including salmon, trout, tuna, herring, and sardines. Omega-3 fatty acids have the ability to alter the activity of neurotransmitters that control mood, motivation, and reward, including dopamine and serotonin, as well as aid in the development and maintenance of brain cell structure and function. Additionally, oxidative stress and inflammation in the brain, which are linked to depression and cognitive loss, can be lessened by omega-3 fatty acids. According to studies, consuming fatty fish or taking fish oil supplements can lessen the signs and symptoms of bipolar disorder, depression, and anxiety, as well as postpone or stop the onset of dementia and Alzheimer's disease.

berries: Antioxidants, including anthocyanins, flavonoids, and polyphenols found in berries—such as blueberries, strawberries, raspberries, and blackberries—can shield the brain from inflammation and oxidative damage. Additionally, berries can promote the development of new brain cells and improve communication between existing ones, all of which can enhance cognitive function, memory, and learning. Additionally, berries can increase dopamine and serotonin synthesis, which can improve mood and lessen stress. Research has indicated that consuming berries or berry extracts can help individuals with depression, anxiety, and cognitive impairment, as well as healthy adults, by improving mood, cognition, and mental health.

Nuts: Nuts that are high in fiber, protein, antioxidants, and good fats are a great source of nutrients for the brain. Examples of these are cashews, walnuts, pistachios, and almonds. Omega-3s and omega-6s, which are important fatty acids that support the construction and function of brain cells and membranes, can be found in nuts. Nuts can also contain vitamin E, zinc, selenium, and magnesium, which can guard against oxidative stress and inflammation in the brain and control the release of neurotransmitters that impact mood, thought, and behavior, such as glutamate, serotonin, and dopamine. Research has indicated that consuming nuts or nut supplements can help patients with depression, anxiety, and cognitive impairment, as well as healthy adults with their mood, memory, attention, and mental health.

Dark chocolate: Dark chocolate is a tasty and healthy treat for the brain, especially when it has a high percentage of cocoa. Theobromine, caffeine, and flavonoids found in dark chocolate can promote the release of endorphins, which are the body's natural mood enhancers and painkillers, as well as improve blood flow to the brain and neurotransmitter function. Additionally, dark chocolate can raise feelings of happiness by increasing dopamine and serotonin and lowering the stress hormone cortisol. Research has indicated that consuming dark chocolate or supplementing with cocoa can enhance mood, mental health, and cognitive function in both healthy individuals and patients suffering from melancholy, anxiety, and cognitive impairment.

Green tea: Popular and healthful, green tea can improve mood and cognitive function. Caffeine, L-theanine, and catechins found in green tea work together to promote blood flow to the brain, improve neurotransmitter and brain cell function, and regulate nervous system activity. Additionally, green tea might lessen oxidative stress and inflammation in the brain, both of which can exacerbate depression and cognitive impairment. Research has indicated that consuming green tea or its extracts can enhance mood, mental health, and cognitive function in both healthy individuals and patients suffering from depression, anxiety, and cognitive impairment.

Our mental and emotional well-being can be greatly influenced by the foods we eat. Certain meals contain healthy nutrients, antioxidants, and phytochemicals that can improve the health and function of our brains. We can obtain a happy mind and a healthier body by increasing our intake of foods that can improve our mood, such as fatty fish, berries, almonds, dark chocolate, and green tea.

4. The Power of Herbs and Spices for Relaxation and Well-Being

Spices and herbs are not only tasty but also extremely potent. They have been utilized for ages to improve health and wellness in a variety of countries and traditions. Certain herbs and spices are particularly good for relaxation and overall health since they can ease mental tension, lower blood pressure, and increase happiness. Here are a few of the best herbs and spices to incorporate into your diet for relaxation and overall health.

Lavender. A fragrant member of the mint family is lavender. Because it can lower blood pressure, heart rate, and levels of the stress hormone cortisol, it has a calming and soothing effect on the nervous system. In addition to lowering anxiety and depression, lavender helps lengthen and enhance sleep. Lavender oil can be used in aromatherapy; dried lavender flowers can be added to tea; or lavender buds can be sprinkled on salads or yogurt. Chamomile. For generations, people have utilized chamomile, a flower that resembles a daisy, as a natural cure for a variety of illnesses. It can relax muscles, alleviate pain, and reduce swelling, giving it a modest sedative and anti-inflammatory effect. In addition to enhancing mood and cognitive performance, chamomile can reduce the incidence of dementia and depression. Before going to bed, you can make chamomile tea, add chamomile extract to your bath, or moisturize your skin with chamomile cream. The root is ginger. The brilliant yellow spice known as turmeric is derived from the roots of the Curcuma longa plant. It is frequently used in Indian cooking and has a flavor that is earthy and toasty. Curcumin, a substance with strong anti-inflammatory and antioxidant qualities, is found in turmeric. Neurotransmitters that control mood, motivation, and reward, such as dopamine and serotonin, can have their activity modulated by curcumin. Additionally, curcumin can shield the brain from inflammation and oxidative stress, both of which can worsen depression and cognitive impairment. Turmeric powder can be taken as a supplement or added to smoothies, soups, and curries.

Saffron. The stigma of the Crocus sativus flower yields the priceless spice of saffron. It is frequently used to color and flavor foods like paella, risotto, and biryani because of its rich and aromatic flavor. Because saffron can raise dopamine and serotonin levels in the brain, it has antidepressant and anti-anxiety properties. In addition to enhancing memory and learning, saffron can postpone or prevent the onset of dementia and Alzheimer's disease. You can add saffron to your food using threads or powder, or you can take saffron supplements.

Ginger. Ginger is a pungent and spicy root that shares a family with turmeric. Due to its ability to enhance blood circulation, digestion, and immunity, it has a warming and energizing effect on the body. Ginger can help lower blood sugar and cholesterol levels, as well as discomfort, inflammation, and nausea. Because ginger raises serotonin and dopamine levels in the brain, it can also improve mood and cognitive function. You can take ginger supplements or add fresh or dried ginger to your juice, tea, or stir-fries.

Spices and herbs can have a significant effect on wellbeing and relaxation. They can shield the brain from harm and illness and aid in mental relaxation, stress reduction, and happiness promotion. Increase your intake of herbs and spices to take advantage of their flavorful and healthful effects.

5.The Importance of Hydration and How to Drink More Water

Since water makes up over 60% of the human body and is crucial to numerous biological processes, it is necessary for life as we know it. But a lot of individuals don't drink enough water to stay hydrated, which can cause several health issues like kidney stones, exhaustion, migraines, and dehydration, among other things. Consequently, it's critical to comprehend the advantages of staying hydrated and learn how to increase your daily water intake.

Among the advantages of being hydrated are:

- It aids in controlling blood pressure, digestion, and body temperature.
- It prevents dryness and irritation by lubricating the skin, eyes, and joints.

By eliminating waste products and poisons from the body, it lowers the chance of illness and infection.

- It strengthens the mood, the brain, and the immune system, improving mental and emotional health.
- It guards against dehydration, which can result in symptoms including dry mouth, thirst, lightheadedness, disorientation, and fainting.
- Among the strategies to increase water intake are:
- Always have a reusable water bottle on you, and fill it up frequently.

- On your computer or phone, set alarms or reminders to remind you to drink water regularly.
- Before, during, and after meals and snacks, sip water.

Use cucumbers, fruits, or herbs to flavor your water.

Consume foods high in water content, such as salads, soups, fruits, and vegetables.

Swap out sugary beverages like soda, juice, and coffee for herbal tea or water. You may boost your water intake and reap the benefits of hydration by using these suggestions. Recall that water is a source of happiness and health in addition to being a requirement.

6. The Effects of Caffeine, Alcohol, and Sugar on Your Mood

Three typical chemicals that many individuals use regularly are sugar, alcohol, and caffeine. They can affect the body and brain in several ways, including mood. I'll touch on each of these drugs' potential beneficial and harmful effects on mood in this post.

One stimulant that can improve alertness, energy, and mental function is caffeine. Additionally, it might elevate mood and encourage productivity. But caffeine can also be detrimental to mood, particularly if taken excessively or by those who are sensitive to its effects. Irritability, anxiety, jitters, sleeplessness, and depression are all related to caffeine consumption. Additionally, it may cause blood sugar to rise and plummet, exacerbating mood swings, cravings, and stress. Additionally, caffeine can disrupt the quantity and quality of sleep, which can have an impact on mood the following day. Headaches, exhaustion, and depressed moods are among the mood disorders that can result from caffeine addiction and withdrawal. Alcohol is a depressant that lowers tension, anxiety, and inhibitions. Additionally, it can improve leisure, relaxation, and social relations. But alcohol can also be detrimental to one's mood, particularly if it's ingested excessively or by someone who is already vulnerable. Alcohol usage can lead to mood disorders, violence, rage, and hostility. Additionally, it may impede decision-making, memory, and judgment. Additionally, alcohol may disrupt the proper ratio of neurotransmitters in the brain, including dopamine and serotonin, which may have an impact on mood. In addition to causing hangovers and sleep cycle disruption, alcohol can also hurt mood the next day. Tremors, convulsions, and delirium are examples of mood disorders that can result from alcoholism and withdrawal.

One type of carbohydrate that can provide you with energy, contentment, and comfort is sugar. Additionally, it can trigger the production of dopamine and endorphins, which can elevate mood and increase reward. But sugar can also be detrimental to mood, particularly if overindulged in or ingested by sensitive people. Blood sugar rises and crashes brought on by sugar can exacerbate mood swings, cravings, and stress. Moreover, sugar can lead to insulin resistance, oxidative stress, and inflammation, all of which can have an impact on mood and the brain. Additionally, sugar may disrupt the proper ratio of neurotransmitters in the brain, including dopamine and serotonin, which may have an impact on mood. In addition to causing headaches, irritation, and low mood, sugar addiction and withdrawal can also lead to mood disorders.

Sugar, alcohol, and caffeine can all affect mood in different ways, both favorably and unfavorably. Numerous variables, including quantity, frequency, timing, and individual variances, affect the effects. Consequently, it's critical to understand how these medications impact mood and to use them sparingly and sensibly.

Chapter 3

How to Plan and Prepare Healthy Meals and Snacks

One of the best methods to enhance your health and well-being is to eat nutritious meals and snacks. Nonetheless, a lot of people find it difficult to find the drive, time, and energy to organize and cook wholesome meals. Here are some pointers to help you get past these obstacles and have a balanced, healthy diet.

- Make advance plans. You may save time, money, and stress by organizing your meals and snacks for the coming week. To plan your meals for breakfast, lunch, supper, and snacks, use meal-planning software, a calendar, or a notebook.

To ensure that the recipes you select meet your dietary requirements and preferences, you can also review the nutrition facts and ingredient lists. Making a list and sticking to it will also help you avoid impulsive purchases and costly, unhealthy eating out.

- Create a list of groceries. Make a list of the foods and ingredients you need to buy based on your meal plan. This will make your shopping more productive and help you stay away from unneeded or unhealthy purchases. Your list can also be arranged into categories like fruits, vegetables, grains, dairy products, proteins, and snacks. Aim to follow your list; otherwise, you may find yourself lured by processed foods and junk food as you peruse the aisles.

- Purchase wisely. Try to get the majority of whole, fresh, and minimally processed foods when you shop at the grocery store. While packaged and processed foods are typically available in the central aisles of the store, these foods are typically located around the store's perimeter. Select a range of fruits and vegetables that are high in fiber, vitamins, minerals, and antioxidants, as well as different colors, textures, and flavors. Choose whole grains that are high in fiber, complex carbs, and other nutrients, such as brown rice, oats, and whole wheat bread. Choose low-fat or fat-free dairy products, such as milk, yogurt, and cheese, which give calcium, protein, and other nutrients; choose lean proteins, such as chicken, turkey, fish, eggs, beans, and nuts;

they are necessary for the development and repair of muscles, organs, and tissues. Reduce your consumption of sodium, added sugars, trans fats, and saturated fats, as these can raise your chance of developing chronic illnesses like diabetes, obesity, and heart disease.

- Prepare in advance. You can save time and hassle during the week by preparing some of your meals and snacks in advance. Foods like soups, stews, casseroles, salads, and cereals can be prepared in large quantities and frozen or refrigerated for later use. Fruits and vegetables can also be chopped, sliced, or diced, then stored for convenient access in bags or airtight containers. For convenience, you may also split out your snacks, including crackers, granola bars, nuts, and dried fruits, and store them in tiny containers or ziplock bags. Planning can also help you avoid overindulging or skipping meals, as well as limit your calorie intake and portion sizes.

- Have pleasure in your food. nourishing meals and snacks are good for your body, mind, and soul. Make sure you are eating enough of these. Eating ought to be enjoyable and fulfilling, rather than a duty or a penalty. Aim to eat consciously, which entails observing your body's signals of hunger and fullness, enjoying the tastes and textures of your food, and putting away electronic devices like phones, computers, and TVs. You can eat less, feel fuller, and appreciate your meal more when you eat with awareness. Sharing meals and snacks with loved ones, friends, or coworkers, as well as experimenting with new dishes, cuisines, and ingredients, may all add to the enjoyment and social aspect of eating.

You may plan and make nutritious meals and snacks that will feed your body, mind, and spirit by using the advice in this article. Recall that maintaining a nutritious diet is a way of life, not a diet. Moderation is key; deprivation is not the answer. It is about growth, not perfection. The little adjustments you make now can have a major impact on your health and well-being. Salutations.

7.How to Mindfully Eat and Enjoy Your Food

One of the most fundamental human activities is eating. That being said, a lot of individuals don't think about what, how, when, where, or why they consume. They might eat things that don't nourish their bodies and minds, or they might eat too quickly, too much, or too little. In addition to hunger, they could eat due to boredom, stress, or emotion. These behaviors can result in weight issues, poor health, and discontentment with food and life in general.

People who practice mindful eating can overcome these negative eating habits and cultivate a happier, more positive connection with food. The foundation of mindful eating is mindfulness, which is acceptance and curiosity about the current moment. Making conscious decisions that promote one's health and well-being while eating entails being aware of the feelings, ideas, and sensations that come up before, during, and after meals.

The advantages of mindful eating are numerous and include:

- enhancing metabolism and digestion through mindful eating and proper chewing
- Using the senses to experience and appreciate food more fully by observing its flavors, textures, colors, and scents
- controlling hunger and appetite by paying attention to your body's cues and just consuming food until you're full, not overstuffed.
- identifying and managing the emotional and environmental triggers that lead to thoughtless

eating to reduce overeating and binge eating
- Avoiding criticism and judgment of oneself and one's dietary decisions might help one become more self-aware and compassionate.
- encouraging healthy eating practices by selecting wholesome, delectable, and filling foods

One can take the following easy steps to practice mindful eating:
- Take a moment to consider your motivations for eating before you eat. Are you bored, anxious, upset, hungry, or thirsty? If you're not hungry, find something else to eat or drink, go for a stroll, or have a conversation with a buddy.
- Pick a spot to dine that is both cozy and devoid of distractions, such as the TV, phone, or computer. To unwind and center yourself, take a

few deep breaths while sitting
down.

- Observe the food on your plate as
  you eat. Take note of the food's
  hues, forms, and aromas. Give
  thanks to your meal for providing
  you with nourishment and energy.
- Eat them in tiny portions and chew
  them well. Savor every bite's flavor
  and texture. In between mouthfuls,
  set down your utensils and
  periodically sip on some water.
- Pay attention to your body and your
  emotions when you eat. What is
  your mood after eating? Are you
  finding it enjoyable? Do you feel
  satisfied, or are you still hungry?
  Not when the platter is empty, but
  rather when you are satisfied, stop
  eating.

Observe your bodily and emotional state
after eating. Do you feel content, joyful,
energized, or drowsy? What is the feeling

in your stomach? What affects your mood? Think back on your dining experience and the lessons you took away.

You can change the way you feel about food and yourself by engaging in mindful eating practices. You may nourish your body, mind, and spirit by eating with joy, gratitude, and awareness. You will also learn that eating is really about thriving as opposed to just surviving.

8.How to Deal with Cravings and Emotional Eating

Emotional eating and cravings are frequent obstacles faced by many individuals trying to eat better and reduce their weight. Strong desires to consume particular foods, typically rich in sugar, fat, or salt, are known as cravings. Eating for emotions other than physical hunger, such as stress, boredom, grief, or rage, is known as emotional eating. Emotional eating and cravings can undermine your health objectives and leave you feeling angry and guilty.

To recover control over your eating patterns and deal with cravings and emotional eating, there are strategies available. The following advice will help you manage:

- Determine your stressors. The first step is to identify the triggers that lead to your emotional eating or food cravings. You can record what you eat when you eat, how you feel, and what makes you want to eat in a food and mood journal. This can assist you in identifying trends and determining the circumstances, feelings, or ideas that trigger your desire to eat. For instance, you might see that, in moments of stress or boredom, you need chocolate or chips.

- Look for healthier substitutes. Knowing your triggers will help you deal with them more healthily than by grabbing food. For instance, you can attempt some relaxation methods like deep breathing, yoga, or meditation if you have a sweet tooth when you're stressed out. You can find interesting hobbies or pastimes, like reading, painting, or gardening if you eat when you're bored. You can get support and consolation from a friend, family member, or therapist if you eat when you're depressed.

- Take a break. Distracting yourself until the craving or emotional need to eat passes is sometimes the best approach to dealing with it. You can attempt to distract yourself from food by doing anything else when you have a want, as they typically only last a few minutes. You may play a game, go on a stroll, watch a hilarious video, listen to music, or call a friend. Your appetite or urge may have subsided by the time you're done.
- Eat with awareness. Eating with awareness of your body and food while avoiding criticism or

judgment is known as mindful eating. You can eat less, feel fuller after eating, and appreciate your meal more when you eat mindfully. You can take the following actions to engage in mindful eating:

1.Determine your level of hunger and your motivation for eating before you eat. Do you feel emotionally or physically hungry? Try to find another means to satisfy your emotional demands if you're not physically hungry, as previously suggested.

2. Select a quiet area away from distractions like the TV, phone, or internet when you are eating. Place your utensils down once you've sat down and taken a few bites of your meal. Pay attention to the food's flavor, texture, aroma, and presentation. Chew gently, enjoying every taste.

3. Pay attention to your body and your emotions when you eat. What is your

mood after eating? Are you finding it enjoyable? Do you feel satisfied, or are you still hungry? Not when the platter is empty, but rather when you are satisfied, stop eating.

4. Observe your bodily and emotional state after   eating. Do you feel content, joyful, energized, or   drowsy? What is the feeling in your stomach? What affects your mood? Think back on your dining experience and the lessons you took away.

- Treat yourself with kindness. It's difficult to control urges and emotional eating, and you might not always be successful. It's common to make mistakes and eat things you hadn't intended to. Nonetheless, attempt to treat oneself with kindness and compassion rather than punishing and feeling bad about yourself. Recall that, despite your best efforts, you are a human. Go forward and learn from your blunders. Don't allow one failure to derail your motivation or your development. There's always the option to restart and try again.

You may better manage your connection with food and yourself by implementing these strategies for managing cravings and emotional eating. Along with reaching your health objectives, you might also feel happier and more confident. Recall that eating is both a joy and a necessity. As long as you eat sensibly and in moderation, you can enjoy your meal without feeling guilty or regretful. It's possible to manage your emotions in other ways besides turning to food as a crutch. It is within your ability and choice to lead a healthy diet and lifestyle.

9.How to Create a Positive and Supportive Food Environment

A food environment that is encouraging and supportive respects each person's needs and preferences, promotes a positive relationship with food and supports healthy eating habits. Your physical, mental, and emotional health can all be enhanced by creating a welcoming and encouraging eating environment. The following advice will assist you in establishing a welcoming and encouraging food environment in your house, place of employment, school, or community:

Make wholesome food easily accessible. Increasing the accessibility and visibility of nutritious foods is one of the simplest ways to eat a better diet. To do this, fill your freezer, refrigerator, and pantry with a wide range of nutrient-dense foods, including whole grains, fruits, vegetables, lean meats, low-fat dairy, nuts, seeds, and legumes. Additionally, you can make a few nutritious meals and snacks in advance and keep them in portion-sized bags or containers for convenient access. You can pack a healthy lunch and snacks for work or school, or you can choose one of the nutritious selections from the cafeteria or vending machine. You can help your neighborhood's farmers' markets, community gardens, or food co-ops by supporting them if they offer reasonably priced, fresh produce. Establish a comfortable and laid-back dining environment. Eating should not be a stressful or hurried activity, but rather one that is joyful and communal. Setting the table, shutting off the TV, phone, and internet, and having uplifting and meaningful talks with your loved ones, friends, or coworkers can all help to create a comfortable and laid-back dining environment. In addition, you can use candles, play some relaxing music, and adorn the table with flowers or plants. Eating in a comfortable and laid-back setting encourages conscious eating, food savoring, and increased satisfaction. Value and honor uniqueness and diversity. When it comes to food and eating, everyone has various demands, preferences, tastes, and objectives. You can appreciate and honor variety and uniqueness by not placing pressure, judgment, or criticism on yourself or other people because of their dietary preferences. You can also try new foods or recipes that pique your curiosity and be observant and inquisitive about various foods, cuisines, and cultures. In addition, you can accept and value the distinctions between the forms, dimensions, and functionalities of your own and other people's bodies without drawing comparisons or making judgments about them. Developing a healthy body image, self-esteem, and self-compassion can be facilitated by acknowledging and appreciating variation and individuality.

Ask for help and direction when you need it. It can be difficult at times to create a welcoming and encouraging food environment, particularly when dealing with obstacles like eating disorders, health issues, food allergies, or food insecurity. In these situations, you might need to look for advice and direction from experts, such as dietitians, physicians, therapists, or counselors, who can assist you in addressing your unique requirements and difficulties. In addition, you can turn to your community, friends, or family for help and advice. They can offer you material, practical, or emotional support. Reaching out for assistance and direction when required can help you get over challenges, manage stress, and accomplish your objectives.

You may improve your health and happiness by creating a positive and encouraging eating environment by using the advice in this article. Recall that fostering a welcoming and encouraging eating environment is an ongoing effort that calls for awareness, intention, and action. You can begin right now and implement little adjustments that will have a significant impact on your life.

Chapter 4

How to Track Your Food and Mood Journal.

By keeping a food and mood journal, you can monitor your consumption of food and beverages as well as your emotional state before, during, and following meals and snacks. It can improve your overall health and well-being, assist you in identifying any dietary sensitivity, and increase your awareness of your eating patterns.

Start a food and mood journal by doing the following:

Choose a format based on what you require. You can use any method—an app, a spreadsheet, or a notebook—that is easy to use and handy for you.

Keep a journal of everything you eat, including the type, amount, time, and place. Give as much detail as you can about your eating experience, including who you were with, what you were doing, and how you were feeling, as these factors may have an impact on the meals you select.

Before and after each meal or snack, rate your level of hunger and fullness on a scale of 1 to 10, where 1 is extremely hungry and 10 is very full. Acquiring an understanding of your body's signals might help you avoid overeating or undereating.

Before, during, and after each meal or snack, write down your thoughts and emotions using words, emojis, or any other technique that suits you best. You can also note any thoughts or feelings that come up with food, like cravings, guilt, contentment, or pleasure.

When you go through your journal regularly, look for any patterns, trends, or connections between your eating and drinking patterns and your emotional condition. You may find that certain foods or drinks make you feel better or worse, or that your emotions affect what you choose to consume. Equipped with this understanding, you can make choices that enhance your pleasure and overall health.

The following advice can help your food and mood journals function more effectively:

Be accurate and sincere. Don't change or remove any information to present yourself in a better or worse light. The purpose of the journal is to help you better understand yourself, not to criticize yourself.

Be loyal and dependable. Try to write in your journal every day as much as you can. The more data you have, the more insights you can get.

Be open-minded and curious. You can't pretend to be an authority on your eating patterns or feelings. You might discover something new or surprising that improves your relationship with food and yourself.

10. How to Balance Your Macronutrients and Micronutrients

Your health and wellness must maintain a balance between macronutrients and micronutrients. Macronutrients, which include lipids, proteins, and carbs, are the nutrients that provide you with energy. The vitamins and minerals known as micronutrients help your body perform a variety of tasks, including growth, metabolism, and immunity.

You must take into account your unique demands, objectives, and tastes to balance your macronutrient intake. Generally speaking, you should get 20%–35% of your calories from fats, 10%–35% from proteins, and 45%–65% from carbohydrates. Nevertheless, based on your exercise level, body composition, medical issues, and food preferences, you might need to modify these ratios.

You must consume a range of foods from several dietary groups, including fruits, vegetables, grains, dairy, meat, and legumes, to maintain a balance of micronutrients. Different kinds of micronutrients that assist your health are found in each food group. For instance, vitamin C, which supports collagen synthesis and your immune system, is abundant in fruits and vegetables. Dairy products and grains are excellent providers of calcium, which fortifies teeth and bones. Iron is found in meat and beans, and it aids in the oxygenation of your blood.

It could be more difficult to obtain some micronutrients from food alone if you have dietary restrictions or adhere to a particular eating schedule. If so, you might need to take supplements to get the micronutrients you need. However, before taking any supplements, you should always speak with your doctor because certain micronutrients can be dangerous if taken in excess.

You may attain the best possible health and wellness by striking a balance between your macronutrients and micronutrients. You can make sure that you are getting adequate amounts of both kinds of nutrients to support your body's activities and functions by maintaining a varied and balanced diet.

11.How to Incorporate Superfoods and Supplements into Your Diet

Superfoods are nutrient-dense meals that include advantageous substances that may enhance your overall health and well-being. Products with concentrated levels of vitamins, minerals, herbs, or other ingredients that can enhance your diet are called supplements. You can begin incorporating superfoods and supplements into your diet by replacing some of your current dietary staples with nutrient-dense options. You can swap out white bread for whole-grain bread, white rice for quinoa, and vegetable oil for coconut oil, for instance. Superfoods can also be included in your cuisine by adding nuts, seeds, berries, or spices to your smoothies, cereals, yogurt, and salads. Depending on your needs and preferences, supplements can be taken as liquids, candies, tablets, capsules, powders, or powders. To ensure that supplements are safe and suitable for you, you should speak with your physician or a qualified dietician before using any.

12. How to Optimize Your Circadian Rhythm and Sleep Quality

Your circadian rhythm, which is regulated by temperature, light, and other environmental cues, is your body's natural 24-hour cycle of waking and sleeping. Your energy, mood, digestion, and numerous other body processes are all impacted. Your general health and well-being can be enhanced, and numerous health issues can be avoided, by maintaining a regular and healthy circadian rhythm.

However, a variety of variables, including jet lag, shift work, stress, or irregular sleeping patterns, might interfere with your circadian rhythm. You may suffer from insomnia, excessive daytime sleepiness, weariness, irritability, mood swings, difficulty concentrating, and an elevated risk of chronic illnesses when your circadian rhythm is out of whack.

Thankfully, there are a few easy and efficient methods to improve the quality of your sleep and your circadian rhythm. Here are some pointers to remember: During the day, expose oneself to bright light. Your circadian rhythm is mostly regulated by light, which informs your brain of when to be up and when to go to sleep. You can feel happier, more aware, and more energized during the day if you get enough artificial or natural light. Additionally, it helps facilitate more rapid and restful sleep at night.

Keep the blue light away at night. Electronic gadgets, including LED lights, PCs, TVs, and cellphones, emit blue light. It can block the release of melatonin, the hormone that controls your sleep cycle, and deceive your brain into believing that it is still daytime. This may make it more difficult for you to go to sleep, stay asleep, and have restful sleep. Use blue light-blocking glasses, filters, or apps, or restrict your exposure to blue light at least two hours before bed to prevent this.

Maintain a consistent sleep routine. Maintaining a consistent sleep schedule can assist your circadian rhythm in adjusting to your chosen sleep pattern. You can also benefit from this by getting the seven to nine hours of sleep that most adults require each night. Aim to avoid taking naps during the day, particularly in the late afternoon or evening, as this may disrupt your sleep at night.

Establish a cozy and tranquil sleeping space. Ensure that your bedroom is cool, quiet, dark, and cozy. To keep out outside light, cover your eyes with an eye mask, drapes, or blinds. To block out distracting noises, use earplugs, a fan, a white noise machine, or other equipment. Set the temperature of your clothes, bedding, and thermostat so that it is comfortable. Avoid coffee, alcohol, nicotine, and heavy meals before bed. - Use aromatherapy, meditation, music, or other relaxation techniques to calm your mind and body before bed. These drugs have the ability to elevate blood pressure and heart rate, excite the neurological system, and impair the quality of sleep. Avoid consuming coffee, tea, energy drinks, or other caffeinated beverages in the late afternoon or evening, as caffeine can remain in your system for up to six hours. Although alcohol can initially make you feel drowsy, it can also interfere with your sleep cycles, increase your frequency of waking, and decrease your quality of deep, dreamless sleep—a critical stage of sleep for memory and learning. Nicotine is a stimulant that might impede your ability to fall asleep and keep you awake. Overindulging in food might result in heartburn, acid reflux, or indigestion, all of which can disrupt your sleep. Three hours before going to bed, try not to eat or drink anything; instead, have a little snack or some herbal tea.

Chapter 5

How to Manage Stress and Anxiety with Mindfulness and Meditation

In the fast-paced and demanding world of today, stress and anxiety are prevalent issues that many individuals deal with. They may impede our ability to be productive, happy, and healthy. Thankfully, there are practical strategies for handling stress and anxiety, and mindfulness and meditation are two of them.

Being mindful involves focusing attention on the here and now without bias or diversion. The practice of meditation involves concentrating attention on a single thing, like the breath, a word, or a sound. By breaking the pattern of unfavorable thoughts and feelings that frequently precede stress and anxiety, mindfulness and meditation can assist us in lowering these feelings.

For stress and anxiety, some advantages of mindfulness and meditation include:

- They can assist us in lowering blood pressure, heart rate, blood sugar, and nervous system calmness—all of which are frequently heightened by stress and anxiety.
- They can assist us in becoming more conscious of our thoughts, emotions, and physical sensations, as well as in learning to accept them without attempting to alter or respond to them.
- They can lessen the propensity to condemn, blame, or avoid ourselves or our issues and assist us

in cultivating a more upbeat and sympathetic attitude toward ourselves and others.

- Instead of acting impulsively or defensively in difficult situations, they can help us improve our resilience and coping abilities and help us respond to stressful situations in a more positive and values-consistent way.
- They can assist us in enhancing our well-being and mood as well as preventing or lowering the risk of depression, which is frequently associated with stress and worry.

Mindfulness and meditation can be applied in a variety of ways, according to one's needs and preferences. Several of the typical techniques are.

- Mindfulness-based stress reduction, or MBSR, is an eight-week therapy method that consists of daily mindfulness activities to practice at home and weekly group workshops. Through yoga and meditation, MBSR teaches people how to become more mindful.

- Cognitive-behavioral therapy (CBT) and mindfulness-based cognitive therapy (MBCT) are two therapeutic approaches that are used to treat depression. By teaching individuals how to identify and break free from the negative thought patterns that lead to depression, MBCT helps people avoid relapsing into depression.

- A quick and easy method to practice mindfulness on your own at any time or location is through mindfulness meditation. To begin, locate a peaceful and comfortable area and set a timer for a few minutes. After that, you can concentrate on your breathing and pay attention to how it feels to inhale and exhale. Remind yourself to breathe whenever your mind strays from it, without passing judgment on your thoughts or yourself. Once you gain comfort and confidence in your meditation sessions, you can progressively extend their length and frequency.

- Exercises that promote mindfulness are a great way to start incorporating mindfulness into your everyday routine and form a habit. Any regular task, like eating, walking, brushing your teeth, or doing the dishes, can be chosen, and it can be completed with complete awareness and focus. Another thing you can do is make an effort to recognize and value the little things in life that make you happy, like a lovely flower, a warm smile, or a tasty meal.

There are no miracle drugs that can make stress and worry go away, nor can mindfulness and meditation. These are abilities that might not be useful to everyone and call for patience and practice. But they have been shown to work for a lot of people, and they can provide a complete, all-natural approach to reducing stress and anxiety and enhancing your quality of life. How about trying them out?

13. How to Boost Your Mood with Physical Activity and Exercise

Exercise and physical activity are beneficial for both your physical and mental well-being. They can elevate your mood, lessen stress, and raise your sense of self-worth. Here are a few ways that

exercise and physical activity might improve your happiness:
They get endorphins out. Natural molecules called endorphins are produced by your body during physical activity. They relieve pain and improve mood, leaving you feeling content and at ease.
They lower cortisol levels. Your body releases the hormone cortisol when you are stressed. Depression, weight gain, and inflammation can all result from it. Exercise and physical activity can reduce cortisol levels and improve your ability to handle stress. 2. They raise serotonin levels. A chemical called serotonin controls your mood, appetite, and sleep patterns. Sleeplessness, anxiety, and despair can be brought on by low serotonin levels. Exercise and physical activity can raise your serotonin levels, which can enhance your mood and general well-being. 3. They enhance how

you see yourself. Exercise and physical activity can improve your appearance, help you tone your muscles, and help you lose weight. This can improve your body image, confidence, and self-esteem. 4. They offer social assistance. Exercise and physical activity can be fantastic ways to socialize, make new friends, and have fun. You can take advantage of the support and companionship of others by joining a fitness class, sports team, or gym.

Depending on your tastes, objectives, and capacity, you can select from a wide variety of physical activities and exercises. Among the typical ones are: aerobic workout. This includes any exercise, including cycling, swimming, dancing, or running, that quickens your breathing and heart rate. Engaging in aerobic exercise can enhance cardiovascular health, burn calories, and lessen anxiety and melancholy. 12.

Strengthening exercises. This includes any workout, including the use of resistance bands, lifting weights, or bodyweight movements like planks, squats, and push-ups. In addition to boosting metabolism, bone density, and muscle mass, strength training can help you avoid accidents and long-term illnesses.

Exercise your flexibility. This includes any type of exercise that stretches your joints and muscles, such as tai chi, pilates, or yoga. Exercises for flexibility can ease pain and stiffness and enhance your range of motion, posture, and balance.

Exercise your balance. This includes any exercise that tests your balance and coordination, like headstands, walking on a beam and one-legged stands. Exercises for balance can increase your mental performance, increase your agility, and prevent falls.

All adults should engage in two days of strength training exercise in addition to 150 minutes of moderate-intensity aerobic exercise or 75 minutes of vigorous-intensity aerobic exercise per week, according to the Department of Health and Human Services. As long as you enjoy and feel comfortable with it, you can begin with smaller amounts and progressively increase the time, frequency, and intensity of your workout. Finding something you enjoy and sticking with it is crucial, and you'll soon see the benefits for your mental and emotional well-being.

14. How to Build Healthy Habits and Stick to Them

Good habits enhance your emotional, mental, or physical health. They can improve your quality of life, increase your energy and mood, and aid in the management or prevention of chronic illnesses. However developing good habits can be difficult, particularly if you have to resist temptations or ingrained behaviors. Here are some pointers for creating and maintaining healthy habits: Begin with a narrow focus. Try not to make all the changes at once. Choose one or two habits that are significant and doable for you, then deconstruct them into explicit, quantifiable activities. For instance, state that you "will eat a fruit or a vegetable with every meal" as opposed to "I want to eat healthier." You can monitor your development and recognize your successes in this way.

Identify your driving force. Consider your motivation for creating a healthy habit as well as the long-term advantages. Put your justifications in writing and post them wherever you can see them, like on your phone, fridge, or mirror. If you find yourself losing motivation or wanting to skip a day, remind yourself why you are doing this.

Establish a schedule. To incorporate your healthy habit into your daily routine, try to perform it at the same time and location each day. For instance, you can work out more in the morning before work or in the evening after supper. In addition, you can utilize cues or triggers—like wearing your workout attire, setting an alarm, or keeping your water bottle close by—to help you remember to engage in your habit.

Make it fun. To help you look forward to practicing your healthy habit, find ways to make it enjoyable and fulfilling. For instance, you can work out, prepare food, or practice meditation while listening to your preferred music, podcast, or audiobook. To encourage one another and spend some social time, you might also extend an invitation to a friend, member of your family, or coworker to come along.

Be understanding and tolerant. Don't count on success or quick fixes. It takes time and work to develop healthy habits, and you will encounter setbacks and difficulties from time to time. Learn from your mistakes and move on, rather than letting shame or discouragement get in the way. Never forget that each day presents a brand-new chance to start over and get back on track.

Conclusion

Now that you've finished the book, maybe you have a better understanding of how eating habits impact mental health. You've also learned a few doable and efficient ways to eat in a way that makes you happier, calmer, and healthier. It's time to put all you've learned into practice and design a customized eating schedule that will help you relax.

The three primary parts of your action plan should be your goals, your activities, and your evaluation. The following is how each component can be made:

Your objectives. Your objectives are the precise, quantifiable results you hope to attain while using food as a calming agent. You might want to lower your stress levels, elevate your mood, sharpen your focus, or increase your vitality, for instance. Depending on your requirements and preferences, you may have one or several goals. Make sure, though, that your objectives are pertinent to your circumstances, reasonable, and achievable. The SMART criterion might assist you in establishing your goals. Time-bound, relevant, quantifiable, achievable, and specific.

What you did. Your activities are the specific, dependable steps you'll take to accomplish your objectives. You could, for instance, adopt an anti-inflammatory diet, limit or stay away from foods that make you anxious or stressed, eat more foods that make you happy and relaxed, use herbs and spices to improve your health, drink more water, cut back on your intake of sugar, alcohol, and caffeine, plan and prepare healthy meals and snacks, eat mindfully and enjoy your food, deal with cravings and emotional eating, and establish a welcoming and encouraging eating environment. Several actions are available to you based on your resources and goals. But make sure what you do is understandable, easy to follow, and achievable. The SMART criterion can also be used to assist you in defining your actions.

Your assessment. The regular, sincere appraisal of your achievements and progress is known as your evaluation. For instance, your assessment might involve keeping tabs on your food intake, keeping an eye on your mental health indicators, measuring the effectiveness of your goals, thinking back on your setbacks and accomplishments, and modifying your strategy as necessary. You can assess your plan using a variety of instruments and techniques, including a self-evaluation, a questionnaire, a scale, a food and mood journal, and feedback forms. Depending on your objectives and course of action, you can review your plan on a daily, weekly, monthly, or quarterly basis. Make sure, nevertheless, that your assessment is factual, truthful, and helpful. The SMART criteria can also be used to assist you in creating your evaluation.

You will be able to eat to boost your mental health and quiet your thoughts by making and adhering to your action plan. Recall that eating to relieve mental stress is a long-term rather than a temporary remedy. It's a lifestyle, not a diet. It is about growth, not perfection. You can begin right now and implement little adjustments that will have a significant impact on your life. It is within your ability and choice to lead a healthy diet and lifestyle.